Who:	Date:

Where:

Activity:

Toys used:

Duration:

Protection used:

STI Test:	Date:

Rating:

( ) ( ) ( ) ( ) ( )

Notes:

Who:	Date:
Where:	
Activity:	
Toys used:	
Duration:	
Protection used:	

STI Test:	Date:

Rating:

Notes:

Who:	Date:

Where:

Activity:

Toys used:

Duration:

Protection used:

STI Test:	Date:

Rating:

Notes:

Who:	Date:
Where:	
Activity:	
Toys used:	
Duration:	
Protection used:	
STI Test:	Date:

Rating:

Notes:

Who:	Date:
Where:	
Activity:	
Toys used:	
Duration:	
Protection used:	

STI Test:	Date:

Rating:

Notes:

Who:	Date:

Where:

Activity:

Toys used:

Duration:

Protection used:

STI Test:	Date:

Rating:

Notes:

Who:	Date:
Where:	
Activity:	
Toys used:	
Duration:	
Protection used:	
STI Test:	Date:

Rating:

○ ○ ○ ○ ○

Notes:

Who:	Date:
Where:	
Activity:	
Toys used:	
Duration:	
Protection used:	
STI Test:	Date:

Rating:

○　○　○　○　○

Notes:

Who:	Date:
Where:	
Activity:	
Toys used:	
Duration:	
Protection used:	
STI Test:	Date:

Rating:

Notes:

Who:	Date:

Where:

Activity:

Toys used:

Duration:

Protection used:

STI Test:	Date:

Rating:

○ ○ ○ ○ ○

Notes:

Who:	Date:

Where:

Activity:

Toys used:

Duration:

Protection used:

STI Test:	Date:

Rating:

○ ○ ○ ○ ○

Notes:

Who:	Date:
Where:	
Activity:	
Toys used:	
Duration:	
Protection used:	
STI Test:	Date:

Rating:

Notes:

Who:	Date:
Where:	
Activity:	
Toys used:	
Duration:	
Protection used:	
STI Test:	Date:

Rating:

Notes:

Who:	Date:
Where:	
Activity:	
Toys used:	
Duration:	
Protection used:	
STI Test:	Date:

Rating:

◯ ◯ ◯ ◯ ◯

Notes:

Who:	Date:

Where:

Activity:

Toys used:

Duration:

Protection used:

STI Test:	Date:

Rating:

Notes:

Who:	Date:
Where:	
Activity:	
Toys used:	
Duration:	
Protection used:	

STI Test:	Date:

Rating:

○ ○ ○ ○ ○

Notes:

Who:	Date:

Where:

Activity:

Toys used:

Duration:

Protection used:

STI Test:	Date:

Rating:

Notes:

Who:	Date:

Where:

Activity:

Toys used:

Duration:

Protection used:

STI Test:	Date:

Rating:

Notes:

Who:	Date:

Where:

Activity:

Toys used:

Duration:

Protection used:

STI Test:	Date:

Rating:

Notes:

Who:	Date:
Where:	
Activity:	
Toys used:	
Duration:	
Protection used:	

STI Test:	Date:

Rating:

Notes:

Who:	Date:

Where:

Activity:

Toys used:

Duration:

Protection used:

STI Test:	Date:

Rating:

○ ○ ○ ○ ○

Notes:

Who:	Date:

Where:

Activity:

Toys used:

Duration:

Protection used:

STI Test:	Date:

Rating:

Notes:

Who:	Date:
Where:	
Activity:	
Toys used:	
Duration:	
Protection used:	
STI Test:	Date:

Rating:

Notes:

Who:	Date:
Where:	
Activity:	
Toys used:	
Duration:	
Protection used:	
STI Test:	Date:

Rating:

○ ○ ○ ○ ○

Notes:

Who:	Date:

Where:

Activity:

Toys used:

Duration:

Protection used:

STI Test:	Date:

Rating:

Notes:

Who:	Date:

Where:

Activity:

Toys used:

Duration:

Protection used:

STI Test:	Date:

Rating:

○ ○ ○ ○ ○

Notes:

Who:	Date:

Where:

Activity:

Toys used:

Duration:

Protection used:

STI Test:	Date:

Rating: 😟 😠 🙂 😋 😍
○ ○ ○ ○ ○

Notes:

Who:	Date:
Where:	
Activity:	
Toys used:	
Duration:	
Protection used:	
STI Test:	Date:

Rating:

Notes:

Who:	Date:
Where:	
Activity:	
Toys used:	
Duration:	
Protection used:	

STI Test:	Date:

Rating:

Notes:

Who:	Date:

Where:

Activity:

Toys used:

Duration:

Protection used:

STI Test:	Date:

Rating:

○ ○ ○ ○ ○

Notes:

Who:	Date:

| Where: | |

| Activity: | |

| Toys used: | |

| Duration: | |

| Protection used: | |

| STI Test: | Date: |

Rating:

Notes:

Who:	Date:
Where:	
Activity:	
Toys used:	
Duration:	
Protection used:	
STI Test:	Date:

Rating:

Notes:

Who:	Date:

Where:

Activity:

Toys used:

Duration:

Protection used:

STI Test:	Date:

Rating:

Notes:

Who:	Date:
Where:	
Activity:	
Toys used:	
Duration:	
Protection used:	

STI Test:	Date:

Rating: 😟 😠 🙂 😋 😍
⚪ ⚪ ⚪ ⚪ ⚪

Notes:

Who:	Date:
Where:	
Activity:	
Toys used:	
Duration:	
Protection used:	
STI Test:	Date:

Rating:

Notes:

Who:	Date:

Where:

Activity:

Toys used:

Duration:

Protection used:

STI Test:	Date:

Rating:

○   ○   ○   ○   ○

Notes:

Who:	Date:

Where:

Activity:

Toys used:

Duration:

Protection used:

STI Test:	Date:

Rating:

Notes:

Who:	Date:
Where:	
Activity:	
Toys used:	
Duration:	
Protection used:	

STI Test:	Date:

Rating:

Notes:

Who:	Date:

Where:

Activity:

Toys used:

Duration:

Protection used:

STI Test:	Date:

Rating:

Notes:

Who:	Date:

Where:

Activity:

Toys used:

Duration:

Protection used:

STI Test:	Date:

Rating:

Notes:

Who:	Date:

Where:

Activity:

Toys used:

Duration:

Protection used:

STI Test:	Date:

Rating:

Notes:

Who:	Date:
Where:	
Activity:	
Toys used:	
Duration:	
Protection used:	
STI Test:	Date:

Rating:

Notes:

Who:	Date:

Where:

Activity:

Toys used:

Duration:

Protection used:

STI Test:	Date:

Rating:

Notes:

Who:	Date:

Where:

Activity:

Toys used:

Duration:

Protection used:

STI Test:	Date:

Rating:

Notes:

Who:	Date:

Where:

Activity:

Toys used:

Duration:

Protection used:

STI Test:	Date:

Rating:

○   ○   ○   ○   ○

Notes:

Who:	Date:

Where:

Activity:

Toys used:

Duration:

Protection used:

STI Test:	Date:

Rating:

Notes:

Who:	Date:
Where:	
Activity:	
Toys used:	
Duration:	
Protection used:	
STI Test:	Date:

Rating: 😟 😒 🙂 😜 😍
○ ○ ○ ○ ○

Notes:

Who:	Date:

Where:

Activity:

Toys used:

Duration:

Protection used:

STI Test:	Date:

Rating:

○ ○ ○ ○ ○

Notes:

Who:	Date:
Where:	
Activity:	
Toys used:	
Duration:	
Protection used:	
STI Test:	Date:

Rating:

○   ○   ○   ○   ○

Notes:

Who:	Date:

Where:

Activity:

Toys used:

Duration:

Protection used:

STI Test:	Date:

Rating:

○ ○ ○ ○ ○

Notes:

Who:	Date:
Where:	
Activity:	
Toys used:	
Duration:	
Protection used:	
STI Test:	Date:

Rating: 😟 😠 🙂 😋 😍
○ ○ ○ ○ ○

Notes:

Who:	Date:
Where:	
Activity:	
Toys used:	
Duration:	
Protection used:	

STI Test:	Date:

Rating:

Notes:

Who:	Date:

Where:

Activity:

Toys used:

Duration:

Protection used:

STI Test:	Date:

Rating:

Notes:

Who:	Date:

Where:

Activity:

Toys used:

Duration:

Protection used:

STI Test:	Date:

Rating:

○ ○ ○ ○ ○

Notes:

Who:	Date:

Where:

Activity:

Toys used:

Duration:

Protection used:

STI Test:	Date:

Rating:

Notes:

Who:	Date:
Where:	
Activity:	
Toys used:	
Duration:	
Protection used:	
STI Test:	Date:

Rating:

Notes:

Who:	Date:

Where:

Activity:

Toys used:

Duration:

Protection used:

STI Test:	Date:

Rating:

Notes:

Who:	Date:
Where:	
Activity:	
Toys used:	
Duration:	
Protection used:	
STI Test:	Date:

Rating:

Notes:

Who:	Date:

Where:	

Activity:	

Toys used:	

Duration:	

Protection used:	

STI Test:	Date:

Rating:

Notes:

Who:	Date:
Where:	
Activity:	
Toys used:	
Duration:	
Protection used:	

STI Test:	Date:

Rating:

Notes:

Who:	Date:

Where:

Activity:

Toys used:

Duration:

Protection used:

STI Test:	Date:

Rating:

○ ○ ○ ○ ○

Notes:

Who:	Date:
Where:	
Activity:	
Toys used:	
Duration:	
Protection used:	

STI Test:	Date:

Rating:

○   ○   ○   ○   ○

Notes:

Who:	Date:

Where:

Activity:

Toys used:

Duration:

Protection used:

STI Test:	Date:

Rating:

Notes:

Who:	Date:

Where:

Activity:

Toys used:

Duration:

Protection used:

STI Test:	Date:

Rating:

Notes:

Who:	Date:

Where:

Activity:

Toys used:

Duration:

Protection used:

STI Test:	Date:

Rating:

Notes:

Who:	Date:

Where:

Activity:

Toys used:

Duration:

Protection used:

STI Test:	Date:

Rating:

Notes:

Who:	Date:
Where:	
Activity:	
Toys used:	
Duration:	
Protection used:	
STI Test:	Date:

Rating:

○　　○　　○　　○　　○

Notes:

Who:	Date:

Where:

Activity:

Toys used:

Duration:

Protection used:

STI Test:	Date:

Rating:

○ ○ ○ ○ ○

Notes:

Who:	Date:
Where:	
Activity:	
Toys used:	
Duration:	
Protection used:	
STI Test:	Date:

Rating:

Notes:

Who:	Date:
Where:	
Activity:	
Toys used:	
Duration:	
Protection used:	
STI Test:	Date:

Rating:

○ ○ ○ ○ ○

Notes:

Who:	Date:
Where:	
Activity:	
Toys used:	
Duration:	
Protection used:	
STI Test:	Date:

Rating:

Notes:

Who:	Date:

Where:

Activity:

Toys used:

Duration:

Protection used:

STI Test:	Date:

Rating:

Notes:

Who:	Date:
Where:	
Activity:	
Toys used:	
Duration:	
Protection used:	
STI Test:	Date:

Rating:

Notes:

Who:	Date:
Where:	
Activity:	
Toys used:	
Duration:	
Protection used:	
STI Test:	Date:

Rating:

Notes:

Who:	Date:

Where:

Activity:

Toys used:

Duration:

Protection used:

STI Test:	Date:

Rating:

◯ ◯ ◯ ◯ ◯

Notes:

Who:	Date:
Where:	
Activity:	
Toys used:	
Duration:	
Protection used:	
STI Test:	Date:

Rating:

○ ○ ○ ○ ○

Notes:

Who:	Date:
Where:	
Activity:	
Toys used:	
Duration:	
Protection used:	
STI Test:	Date:

Rating:

○   ○   ○   ○   ○

Notes:

Who:	Date:

Where:

Activity:

Toys used:

Duration:

Protection used:

STI Test:	Date:

Rating:

Notes:

Who:	Date:
Where:	
Activity:	
Toys used:	
Duration:	
Protection used:	
STI Test:	Date:

Rating:

○ ○ ○ ○ ○

Notes:

Who:	Date:
Where:	
Activity:	
Toys used:	
Duration:	
Protection used:	
STI Test:	Date:

Rating:

Notes:

Who:	Date:

Where:

Activity:

Toys used:

Duration:

Protection used:

STI Test:	Date:

Rating:

○　　○　　○　　○　　○

Notes:

Who:	Date:
Where:	
Activity:	
Toys used:	
Duration:	
Protection used:	
STI Test:	Date:

Rating:

○ ○ ○ ○ ○

Notes:

Who:	Date:
Where:	
Activity:	
Toys used:	
Duration:	
Protection used:	
STI Test:	Date:

Rating:

Notes:

Who:	Date:
Where:	
Activity:	
Toys used:	
Duration:	
Protection used:	

STI Test:	Date:

Rating:

○   ○   ○   ○   ○

Notes:

Who:	Date:
Where:	
Activity:	
Toys used:	
Duration:	
Protection used:	

STI Test:	Date:

Rating: 😕 😠 🙂 😋 😍
○ ○ ○ ○ ○

Notes:

Who:	Date:

Where:

Activity:

Toys used:

Duration:

Protection used:

STI Test:	Date:

Rating:

Notes:

Who:	Date:

Where:

Activity:

Toys used:

Duration:

Protection used:

STI Test:	Date:

Rating:

Notes:

Who:	Date:
Where:	
Activity:	
Toys used:	
Duration:	
Protection used:	

STI Test:	Date:

Rating:	

Notes:

Who:	Date:

Where:

Activity:

Toys used:

Duration:

Protection used:

STI Test:	Date:

Rating:

Notes:

Who:	Date:

Where:

Activity:

Toys used:

Duration:

Protection used:

STI Test:	Date:

Rating:

○ ○ ○ ○ ○

Notes:

Who:	Date:

Where:

Activity:

Toys used:

Duration:

Protection used:

STI Test:	Date:

Rating:

○　○　○　○　○

Notes:

Who:	Date:

Where:

Activity:

Toys used:

Duration:

Protection used:

STI Test:	Date:

Rating:

○ ○ ○ ○ ○

Notes:

Who:	Date:
Where:	
Activity:	
Toys used:	
Duration:	
Protection used:	

STI Test:	Date:

Rating:

Notes:

Who:	Date:

Where:

Activity:

Toys used:

Duration:

Protection used:

STI Test:	Date:

Rating:

○   ○   ○   ○   ○

Notes:

Who:	Date:

Where:

Activity:

Toys used:

Duration:

Protection used:

STI Test:	Date:

Rating:

Notes:

Who:	Date:

Where:

Activity:

Toys used:

Duration:

Protection used:

STI Test:	Date:

Rating:

○ ○ ○ ○ ○

Notes:

Who:	Date:

Where:

Activity:

Toys used:

Duration:

Protection used:

STI Test:	Date:

Rating:

Notes:

Who:	Date:

Where:

Activity:

Toys used:

Duration:

Protection used:

STI Test:	Date:

Rating:

Notes:

Made in the USA
Middletown, DE
02 November 2020